Intermittent Fasting 16:8 Copyright © 2019

Table of Contents

Introduction   4

What Is Intermittent Fasting?   5

   Fed vs. Fasted   6

   Less Feeding, More Fasting   11

   Avoid Carbohydrates   12

   Exercise Helps   12

What Is The 16:8 Fasting?   16

What are the Benefits of 16:8 Intermittent Fasting?   24

Does Fasting Agree With Your Natural Instincts?   29

Best Foods to Eat While Intermittent Fasting   31

   Foods To Avoid   36

Common Mistakes People Make While Intermittent Fasting 37

Tea and Intermittent Fasting: The Perfect Match   41

   Teas That Enhance Intermittent Fasting   43

Intermittent Fasting Myths   47

What Is The Importance of Calories & Macros?   54

How To Determine Calories & Macros   55

Intermittent Fasting FAQ   **60**

Conclusion   **66**

Introduction

Intermittent fasting has become a popular topic both for researchers and health enthusiasts. Intermittent fasting, like the 16:8 fasting, promises weight loss, better performance, increased fat burning and lean muscle preservation.

While there are several different types of Intermittent fasting, like the 5:2 fasting or religious-based fasting, 16:8 is a sustainable pattern that's associated with lean muscle gains. This ebook explores the potential benefits and the best way to determine if Intermittent fasting is right for you.

This manual is for those who;

- Want to learn the basic of intermittent fasting.
- Want a to improve their health.
- Experience a consistent and manageable way to lose weight.
- Want to adhere to a diet and without the hassle of being limited to certain foods.

This manual assumes that you have an exercise program to accompany the fasting program. Maximum fat loss cannot be achieved through diet alone instead it is a combination of exercise and fasting that produces maximum fat loss. If you do not have an exercise program do not fright. An exercise program can be as simply as jogging for 30minutes a day. However it should be noted that a well-designed training program that is tailored towards your goal will produce the best results.

What Is Intermittent Fasting?

The word "Intermittent" is defined as "occurring in irregular intervals". The word fasting is an act in which one refrains from a certain activity for a specific period of time. Simply put Intermittent Fasting is refraining from food for a certain time period. It has two components

- A fasting period: time interval in which you refrain from eating.
- A feeding window: time interval in which you are allowed to eat.

Intermittent fasting has become a popular way to use your body's natural fat-burning ability to lose Intermittent in a short period of time. However, many people want to know, does intermittent fasting work and how exactly does it work? When you go for an extended period of time without eating, your body changes the way that it produces hormones and enzymes, which can be beneficial for Intermittent loss. These are the main fasting benefits and how they achieve those benefits.

Much has been written about Intermittent fasting. Much of it is speculation. Some of it is backed by research. I'm going to do my best to not add to the speculation, but you can broadly break it down into two effects - the effects on your physiology (your body, hormones, etc.), and psychology (your brain). On a physiological level, much of what is going on is at the level of hormones - certain "Intermittent-burning" hormones get up-regulated.

Intermittent fasting has historically been a normal part of life for humans and many organisms. It's a way of tapping into the ancient knowledge that already exists within your biology. Scientists and celebrities alike are popularizing this way of eating. IF is healthy, with benefits from better brain function to protein sparing weight-loss and cancer prevention, and best of all its easy.

Compared to traditional "fasting," fasting is simple and unambiguous. It's always been done. You already unconsciously do it whenever you skip breakfast or dinner. Historically, during hunter-gatherer days, our ancestors were in a fasting state while seeking food. When agriculture was established, civilization came next. But when food was scarce or seasons changed, fasting was still a way of life. Cities and castles stored grain and cured meat for the winter. Before irrigation, lack of rain meant famine, and people fasted to make their stored food last as long as possible until the rains came back and it was possible for crops to survive again.

Religions flourished in this arrangement of people living closer together, sharing and spreading belief and traditions. And religions also prescribed fasting. Hinduism calls fasting "Vaasa" and observes it during special days or festivals, as a personal penance, or to honor their personal gods. Islam and Judaism have Ramadan and Yom Kippur, when it's forbidden to work, eat, drink, wash, wear leather and have intercourse. In Catholicism, it's six weeks of fasting before Easter or before Holy Week

Fed vs. Fasted

Your body is designed to smoothly transition between two different and opposing states: 'fed', and 'fasted'. In the fed state, insulin is elevated, and this signals your body to store excess calories in your fat cells. In the presence of insulin, the burning of fat is halted, while the body burns glucose instead.

In the fasted state, insulin is low (while glucagon and growth hormone, opposing hormones to insulin, are elevated). The body starts mobilizing stored body Intermittent from your fat cells and burning this fat for energy (instead of glucose). The practical importance of all this? You can only burn stored body fat while in the fasted state, and you can only store more body Intermittent while in the fed state.

Unfortunately, over time we seem to be spending less and less of our time in the fasted state and more and more time in the fed state. As a result, our bodies and our cells spend less and less time mobilizing and burning stored body fat for energy, and the glucose-burning pathways are overused.

Eventually, insulin is high all the time and the body avoids burning stored body fat, relying mostly on glucose. Over time, this chronic exposure to so much insulin also leads to 'insulin resistance' where the body secretes even more insulin in response to the fed state. Chronic insulin resistance is the cause of 'metabolic syndrome': obesity, abdominal fat storage, high triglycerides, low HDL or "good" cholesterol, and elevated glucose with eventual type 2 diabetes. 1 in 12 humans on earth currently have full blown type 2 diabetes, while 35% of adults and 50% of older adults have metabolic syndrome, or pre-diabetes.

Someone with insulin resistance is burning predominately glucose on the cellular level, and they rarely ever get the opportunity to burn any body Intermittent. When these people run out of glucose from their last meal, instead of easily transitioning over to the fasted state to burn fat, they become hungry for more glucose as their bodies and cells have decreased capacity for mobilizing and burning Intermittent for energy.

Let's put it this way. Why would a highly obese person ever be hungry? They have enough fat stores to last a very long time. The world record for fasting went to a 456 pound man who fasted for 382 days, consuming only water and vitamins and losing 276 pounds with no ill effects. But the average overweight person is used to being in the fed state, has very little practice in the fasted state, and is continually burning glucose rather than Intermittent at the cellular level. They have insulin resistance, which is both caused by and also leads to chronically high insulin levels, which promotes Intermittent storage and suppresses Intermittent mobilization from the adipocytes. They even have changes in the mitochondria, or tiny energy factories inside the cells. The mitochondria can burn either glucose or fat for fuel, and over time they will have a preference for one over the other; "sugar burners" have increased the pathways in the mitochondria that burn glucose and decreased, or down-regulated, the underused pathway for burning Intermittent. So what happens to the overweight "sugar burner" who stops eating for a few hours? As they run out of glucose from their last meal, instead of seamlessly transitioning to the fasted state and mobilizing and burning stored body fat, they become hungry for more glucose, from carbohydrates! They will spend most of the day trapped in a cycle of eating every few hours, spiking glucose, and then becoming hungry when blood sugar drops.

A good analogy is that of a tanker truck on the freeway filled with oil. If the tanker truck runs out of gas it stops moving, despite the fact that it has 10,000 gallons of potential fuel on board. Why? Because it prefers to run on refined gas and is incapable of burning oil for fuel.

Humans have the ability to become 'fat-adapted' and improve their ability to fuel themselves with stored body fat instead of glucose. However, this takes time and practice, and your body has to do a number of things to slowly up-regulate or increase your intermittent-burning pathways. This includes improving insulin sensitivity to lower insulin and promote Intermittent mobilization into free Intermittentty acids from the adipocytes as well as up-regulating the intermittent-burning pathways at the cellular level (in the mitochondria).

There are several ways to improve 'fat adaptation' or the ability to successfully burn stored body fat for energy, and these include the following:

- Low carbohydrate diets. Eating a LCHF (low carb high fat) diet improves the body's ability to utilize fat for energy rather than glucose, as there is more fat and less glucose available at all times, even in the fed state.
- Exercise. High-intensity exercise depletes glucose and glycogen rapidly, forcing the body to switch over and utilize more Intermittent for fuel. Exercise also improves insulin sensitivity.
- Caloric restriction. Eating fewer calories also equals less glucose available for fuel, so the body is more frequently forced to rely on stored body fat for fuel. You will always naturally eat the lowest calories when you are maximizing nutrient density by eating whole, natural, unprocessed, real foods found in nature.

Intermittent fasting, and spending more time in the fasted state, which gives the body more 'practice' at burning fat. The purpose of this is to highlight intermittent fasting as a strategy for exercising and strengthening the body's ability to exist in the fasted state, burning fat instead of continually burning sugar from the fed state.

Just like anything else, this ability can be strengthened over time with practice. But this ability also atrophies or shrinks over time with lack of use, just like your muscles atrophy when you break your arm and have to wear a cast for weeks. Spending time in the fasted state is actually a form of exercise - a metabolic workout.

In fact, there are a lot of parallels between exercise and fasting. Exercise does all of the following great things:

- Decreases blood glucose.
- Decreases insulin level.
- Increases insulin sensitivity.
- Increases lipolysis and free Intermittentty acid mobilization.
- Increases cellular fat oxidation.
- Increases glucagon (the opposite of insulin).
- Increases growth hormone (the opposite of insulin).

But did you know you can also accomplish all of the above by doing absolutely nothing? The secret is fasting. Extending the amount of time that you spend during your day in the fasted state as opposed to the fed state accomplishes all of these, very similar to exercise. Extending your time in the fasted state is actually a form of metabolic 'exercise', in which you train your body to rapidly and efficiently mobilize free fatty acids from your adipose stores, something you absolutely can get better and better at with the metabolic 'practice' of fasting. Just as overweight and out of shape people struggle to jog or lift weights or participate in other forms of physical exercise, they are also generally out of practice when it comes to rapidly and efficiently mobilizing and burning stored free Intermittentty acids for fuel. Intermittent fasting and spending more of your day in the 'fasted' state and less time in the 'fed' state is a great form of metabolic 'exercise' which has many health benefits, including fat loss.

Less Feeding, More Fasting

One of the best ways to achieve effortless and long-lasting fat loss is to train yourself to eat two meals a day and eliminate snacking. The easiest and best way to accomplish this is to leverage your natural overnight fast by skipping breakfast. No breakfast, lighter lunch, and larger dinner also maximizes the body's natural shifts between sympathetic ("fight or flight") and parasympathetic ("rest and digest") nervous system tone, with higher alertness and activation from sympathetic tone during the day while under-eating, and higher parasympathetic resting tone in the evening during the fed state.

Typically, the fed state starts when you begin eating and for the next three to five hours your body digests and absorbs the food you just ate. Insulin rises significantly, completely shutting off fat-burning and also triggering excess calories to be stored as fat. After the first few hours mentioned above, your body goes into what is known as the post–absorptive state, during which the components of the last meal are still in the circulation. The post - absorptive state lasts until 8 to 12 hours after your last meal, which is when you enter the fasted state. It typically takes 12 hours after your last meal to fully enter the fasted state.

When you're in the fasted state your body can burn fat that has been inaccessible during the fed state. Because we don't enter the fasted state until 12 hours after our last meal, it's rare that our bodies are in this Intermittent burning state. This is one of the reasons why many people who start intermittent fasting will lose fat without changing what they eat, how much they eat, or how often they exercise. Fasting puts your body in a fat burning state that you rarely get to enter during a normal eating schedule.

Avoid Carbohydrates

Eating carbohydrates, especially refined carbohydrates with no fiber, overdrives the 'fed' state, as carbohydrates raise both glucose and insulin higher than other macronutrients (fat, on the other hand, raises glucose and insulin the very least). In general, when you eat a meal, your body spends a few hours processing that food and burning what it can from what you just consumed. Because it has all of this readily available, easy to burn energy in its blood stream, your body will choose to use that as energy rather than the fat you have stored. This is especially true if you just consumed carbohydrates, because these are rapidly converted to glucose and your body prefers to burn sugar as energy before any other source. High glucose is toxic and your body burns extra glucose preferentially to get rid of it, much in the same way that the body burns alcohol consumed for energy prior to other energy calories--alcohol therefore also sabotages intermittent loss.

Exercise Helps

Exercise helps greatly with intermittent adaptation. Your glycogen (the storage form of glucose in your muscles and liver that your body can burn as fuel when necessary) is depleted during sleep and fasting, and will be depleted even further during training, which can further increase insulin sensitivity. This means that a meal immediately following your workout will be stored most efficiently: mostly as glycogen for muscle stores, burned as energy immediately to help with the recovery process, with minimal amounts stored as fat. Compare this to a regular day (no Intermittent fasting). With insulin sensitivity at normal levels, the carbs and foods consumed will see full glycogen stores, enough glucose in the blood stream, and thus be more likely to get stored as fat.

I've identified a few key reasons as to why intermittent fasting for weight loss works so well.

1. Secret Weapon For Battling Cravings

Considering that the mere word "fasting" can make us feel hungry, it's a pleasant surprise for many intermittent fasting followers to discover that, after about 1-2 weeks, they no longer experience any hunger pangs during their fasting windows. And no, it's not just a trick of the mind or extreme willpower. There's a scientific reason why this happens. You see, one of the most important effects that Intermittent fasting has on your body is that your insulin levels become regulated. Instead of rising and falling all day long (which is what happens when you eat all day long), your blood sugar levels stay stable. This automatically translates to less sugar cravings.

The other cool thing that happens when you start intermittent fasting is that the levels of a hormone called "ghrelin" become far more normalized. Ghrelin is known as the hunger hormone. When it's out of whack, that's when you feel hungry all the time. After a couple weeks of intermittent fasting, your ghrelin levels become far more regulated, and that's when your hunger pangs start to disappear.

2. Natural Calorie Restriction, But Better

At the root of nearly every fasting known to man is the concept of calorie restriction. We've all seen the formula:

Calories eaten < calories burned = weight loss

Calorie restriction is also the main reason why most diets fail over the long-term. It goes against human nature and thus is incredibly difficult to sustain.

Intermittent fasting has earned high praise on account of the fact that it naturally leads to calorie restriction, without feeling like that's what you're doing. We like to call it "sneaky" calorie restriction. Here's why: a typical intermittent fasting schedule (eating only between noon and 8:00pm) usually e☐uates to skipping breakfast. Because it's difficult to eat more than a certain number of calories per meal, cutting your day from 3 meals down to 2 can have a noticeable effect over time.

Studies have been done comparing a group of people who were asked to restrict their calories all day, and another group that was asked to follow an Intermittent fasting schedule. Both groups derived similar health benefits, except the Intermittent fasting group experienced better insulin regulation. Most importantly, the intermittent fasting group found their diet much more manageable. For most of us, it's psychologically and biologically easier to restrict our eating to a certain time frame, as opposed to restricting our overall daily caloric intake.

3. Retain Lean Muscle Mass

Perhaps the biggest downside of many restricted calorie diets is that they have been proven to lead to loss of lean muscle mass, which actually slows down your metabolism. This is really bad news for your ability to maintain any weight loss. The good news? Research has shown that intermittent fasting actually helps you retain lean muscle mass while still losing weight.

4. Better Eating Habits

When you intermittent fast, you'll be sticking to a smaller eating window than you're probably used to. This will naturally cut down on late night snacking, which is often a hidden culprit of excess calories and sneaky weight gain. When you know that giving in to the munchies is just going to kick yourself out of fat-burning mode, it's much easier to resist that late-night fridge raid.

5. It's Sustainable

Perhaps one of the most striking things about the Intermittent fasting "craze" is that people are treating it less like a diet and more like a lifestyle. So many followers find themselves not only losing weight, but feeling better and actually wanting to stick with this eating schedule. So Intermittent fasting can quickly become a lifestyle change, as opposed to a crash diet.

What Is The 16:8 Intermittent Fasting?

The 16:8 intermittent fasting fasting limits eating to 8 hours a day and requires fasting for the remaining 16 of 24 hours. Although 16 hours seems like a long time, this includes time spent sleeping. The theory is to wake and work out in a fasted state, which forces your body to draw upon fat stores for energy.

You should consume reasonable meals throughout your 8 eating hours. While fasting, you should drink water, and some choose to include unsweetened tea, coffee, or BCAAs/pre-workout in the mornings before exercise.

Contrary to other intermittent loss methods, the 16:8 intermittent fasting method is not based on hypothetical or personal opinions, but it is based in scientific research. A number of studies conducted in order to investigate the effects of intermittent fasting and some of them included the Leangains protocol of 16 hours of fasting and 8 hours of feeding.

One of the most recent published studies and easily to access for free, was conducted by Moro and her colleagues and investigated the effects of eight weeks of time-restricted feeding on metabolic factors, body composition, strength and other markers in resistance-trained males. The study of Moro and her colleagues compared two groups of resistance trained athletes, the one group used the time-restricted feeding while the other group was on a normal fasting. The first group (time-restricted feeding) consumed their calories in an 8h period of time every day, divided into 3 meals: 1 p.m., 4 p.m. and 8 p.m. The remaining time of the day was the fasting period.

The second group (normal diet) consumed their energy needs divided into 3 meals: 8 a.m., 1 p.m., and 8 p.m. Both groups consumed the same amount of calories and % of macronutrients. In addition, they used a standardized resistance training program. Subjects were tested, before and after the 8 weeks of the program, to compare the results between the 2 groups.

According to the results of the study, the fat mass of the time-restricted feeding group decreased significantly (−16.4 versus a reduction of −2.8 % in the normal fasting group). An increase, similar between the 2 groups was observed on Leg press maximal strength. Insulin and blood glucose levels decreased significantly only in the group of males on the time-restricted feeding.

In addition, triglycerides levels decreased only in the time-restricted feeding group. The hormone adiponectine which is related to increased energy expenditure also was higher only in the time-restricted group. However, anabolic hormone levels, such as testosterone were lower after the time-restricted feeding, while in the normal fasting group no change was observed.

So the scientific research shows that time-restricted feeding maintains muscle mass, reduces body fat levels and inflammation markers. The mechanism of greater fat loss in time-restricted feeding group compared to the normal fasting group seems to be due to the different time of meal distribution. Despite the fact that this study was conducted in resistance trained males, the observation that insulin and blood glucose levels decreased significantly indicates that time-restricted feeding like 16:8 intermittent fasting method could also improve health markers related to patients such as diabetics and obese patients.

Although there is a great number of studies conducted in order to battle obesity and diabetes, very few managed to provide a really effective and useful tool. The 16:8 Intermittent fasting method seems to be a promising natural alternative and future studies are expected to strengthen current scientific findings.

The 16:8 fasting style of Intermittent fasting was designed for people who want the benefits of intermittent fasting without compromising their fitness and/or strength training. Whereas other methods of intermittent fasting focus more on the fasting cycle and less on the specifics of what an individual is eating, Leangains emphasizes proper pre and post workout nutrition. Berkan also goes in depth to explain calorie cycling, macronutrients and meal times.

Here is a basic breakdown of the 16:8 Intermittent fasting protocol:

There is a 16 hour window for fasting each day. The majority of this time is taken up during sleep. For women this is a 14 hour window as women's bodies and metabolisms differ from men's.

There is an 8 hour window for feeding each day. During this time three meals are usually eaten. For women this is a 10 hour window.

Protein intake remains high on all days. On workout days, it is more important to get carbs before fat. On rest days, fat intake tends to be higher. These variables change depending on the gender, age, body fat, activity levels and the goals of an individual.

Workout days start with a medium-sized meal of meat, veggies and fruit. Training is meant to happen within three hours of this first meal. A larger meal can be had post workout.

Rest days involve a lower calorie intake. Carb consumption should be restricted whereas meat and fibrous veggies make up the bulk of the calories eaten on rest days. The first meal of the day is the largest consisting of roughly 40% of the daily calorie intake.

The last meal of the day should involve a slow digesting protein. This maintains a feeling of fullness and ensures that your body has enough amino acids until the next meal to prevent muscle atrophy.

Whole and unprocessed food should be eaten whenever possible. Avoid processed or liquid foods.

The 5 Rules Of Effortless Fasting

Rule One - Use Caffeine Strategically

If you're not currently taking caffeine/coffee during your fasts then you are missing out big time! Caffeine is much more powerful when ingested in the fasted state. Moreover, caffeine serves to enhance many of the effects of fasting. Caffeine stimulates the metabolism, blunts appetite, increases energy levels, elevates fat mobilization and also heightens mental alertness. Not to mention, coffee is associated with plenty of positive health benefits.

That being said, I recommend strictly limiting your caffeine intake to the fasting portion of the day. If you drink plenty of coffee throughout the day, you will become more and more desensitized to the effects of caffeine. This will diminish the hunger blunting and energy boosting effects of caffeine. Reducing caffeine to the fasted state and only the fasted state, makes fasting downright effortless.

My advice is to drink 2 cups of black coffee during the fast and at no other point in the day. If you want a hot beverage later in the day then go with some herbal tea. If you hate black coffee then I recommend sucking it up. Within a few weeks you will grow a fondness for black coffee that will trump just about anything else.

Rule Two - Workout Intelligently

Intermittent fasting workouts should be based off low volume strength training to build strength and muscle. If you want to burn some calories, low intensity walking is your best bet, which has a neutral effect on appetite. Exercising regularly is very important. When your body remains inactive, no amount of dieting or weight loss pills will help you lose weight. Exercise will create a need for energy, which will be provided by the stored Intermittent. Continue with your regular workout routine, or start working out while you are on the 8-hour diet. Walking, jogging, running, rope jumping, aerobics, swimming, biking, playing a sport, dancing, staircase running, climbing, yoga, and strength training will help you lose Intermittent and build muscle mass. Also, make sure you keep moving while you are at school or office. Take the stairs whenever possible, and ditch your automobile and ride a bike.

There's no need for any additional training on top of this, unless of course you're a competitive athlete and need to do skill work for your sport. Drawn out interval sessions, circuit routines and high volume workout sessions will burn a bunch of energy, rendering you ravenous during your fast. Moreover, these forms of training are completely unnecessary in nature and will only serve to retard your progress from your much more important strength and muscle building sessions.

If you want to do additional exercise, it should be light to moderate in nature. In this case I'd recommend focusing on having fun or learning and honing a skill, rather than trying to destroy yourself in the gym. Recreation sports and yoga or martial arts are great options. Some Intermittent fasting exercise I would not recommend is cross fit, p90x and hour long running sessions.

Intermittent fasting is an incredible tool for staying lean, so make use of it. Focus your efforts on building strength and muscle, add some light activity like brisk walking here and there and throw in some short sprints if you feel so inclined. Other than that, well there's more to life than exercising, and trying to do more intense training is only going to hamper your progress.

Rule Three - Strategic Fruit Snacking

If you find yourself getting hungry before your first meal I recommend snacking on a piece of fruit. Fruit is very helpful in the fasted state because it helps to replenish liver glycogen. When liver glycogen levels become depleted from long fasts, a signal is sent to the brain that triggers hunger.

By having a serving of fruit when you get hungry near the end of your fast, you are effectively down regulating hunger signals. Moreover, replenishing liver glycogen helps to shift you back into an anabolic state.

The best time to eat fruit is on a relatively empty stomach, when carbohydrate stores are low. This ensures that the carbs from the fruit are used to replenish depleted liver glycogen stores. After a big meal with carbs, your liver glycogen levels will be relatively topped off. Any additional fruit on top of this will have to be burned for energy or it will get stored as fat.

Therefore, I recommend eating 2-3 servings of fruit per day to stave off hunger and then getting the rest of your carbs from starches like potatoes and rice, which are better at restocking muscle glycogen. I usually have an apple before lunch and dinner and occasionally a banana before bed.

Bananas are higher in glucose so they do a better job at replenishing muscle glycogen than most fruits. Further, bananas stimulate the release of serotonin in the brain, which improves relaxation and helps with sleep. What's more, bananas are a good source of magnesium and potassium, which promotes muscle relaxation, further enhancing sleep.

Rule Four - Eat Big

If you're switching to Intermittent fasting then you're going to have to eat much bigger meals than you're accustomed to. If you don't adjust the size of your meals accordingly, you will be very low in calories and nutrients and hunger will be pronounced during the fast. Alternatively, you will be tempted to snack on junk to get your calories up, which will likely lead to excessive calorie consumption.

When you feel extremely satisfied and filled up while dropping Intermittent, life is pretty damn good! If you're trying to go too low in calories and eating just two modest meals per day, you'll be in too big of a calorie deficit, and your fasts will be pretty brutal. So don't be scared of eating more than what seems reasonable, you have my whole-hearted permission.

Rule Five - Forget About It

Forget about the fact that you're fasting. You don't have to tell the whole world and your pet gold fish how long you've been fasting for. No one cares. Besides, it's not really a big deal. This is how I believe humans should eat anyways, I think it's crazy eating first thing in the morning.

So don't think that you're bending spoons with your mind all of the sudden because you've been fasting for a big chunk of the day. By not thinking about how long you've been fasting for and by not making a big deal about it, it feels completely natural. It takes the effort and will power out of fasting.

What are the Benefits of 16:8 Intermittent Fasting?

It doesn't seem like going for long periods without food would be beneficial for your body, but let me tell you, there's actually ☐uite a long list of them. Following a 16:8 diet is sometimes referred to as "lean gains", building on theory of burning fat and calories while working out in a fasted state. Intermittent fasting has been shown to be effective in limiting calorie intake to reduce Intermittent while still maintaining performance and muscle tissue.

Here's a rundown of some of the benefits of 16:8 Intermittent fasting:

Accelerates Intermittent loss. Not only are you likely naturally consuming fewer calories due to a restricted eating window, but you're also burning stored body fat for fuel.

Improves glucose uptake efficiency and insulin sensitivity. Intermittent fasting helps to increase insulin mediated glucose uptake rates into tissues that can use it for fuel (e.g. muscle). It also helps to decrease/normalize biomarkers (insulin and glucose) associated with chronic diseases.

Normalizes/decreases appetite. When running off of your main energy store, body Intermittent, rather than incoming sugary foods, your body is using a stable and well regulated supply of energy. Intermittent fasting often helps people eat less in the evening, too. This is time of day when our metabolic response to food tends to worse compared to when it's still light out [4]. It may therefore be healthier to increase food consumption during the day when our bodies are better able to metabolize and use energy.

Culls gut microbiota. Although no one knows what a 'healthy microbiota' looks like, fasting initially culls our gut flora, reduces excess gut permeability and increases overall diversity (somewhat counterintuitively maybe). It's analogous to a gardener removing pesky weeds to encourage the growth of their desired flowers.

Improves brain function. It increases BDNF (brain-derived neurotrophic factor), a protein that's involved in learning and memory, helping us make certain brain pathways faster and more efficient.

Recycles faulty mitochondria. Think of mitochondria as the powerhouse of your cells that unavoidably incur damage over-time, becoming less efficient energy producers. During a fasted state when ATP (energy) levels decrease, the body is stimulated to create more and better mitochondria. This means that when food is available it will be 'burned more cleanly'.

Stimulates autophagy. If you've never heard of the term autophagy, it's essentially our bodies way of housekeeping. A lot of our basic cellular processes create waste that has to either be excreted from our bodies or recycled to improve the efficiency and function of our various organelles [9]. Autophagy is part of that sorting process and is always ongoing, but strongly unregulated when fasting.

Reduces/normalizes oxidative stress and inflammation. Intermittent fasting may enhance the body's resistance to oxidative stress and normalize the amount of damaging free radicals our mitochondria face. It also helps to reduce levels of pro-inflammatory cytokines and stimulate anti-inflammatory pathways which are too often under stimulated.

Provides mental clarity. Fat is the most energy-efficient and energy-dense fuel available to our body – making our brains particularly happy! When our small glucose stores are low (they're never empty) the brain is able to function at its best given it's particularly fuel re□uirements. This leaves us mentally more clear and focused.

Improves fitness. Working out in a fasted state can have many positive effects on the body, such as stronger metabolic adaptations (increased training stimulus), higher sensitivity to growth factors (think muscle synthesis) and improved metabolic responses to post-workout meals, crucial for fast recovery. Just a note of caution: we're talking about health here, not world-class athletic performance. So although fasted training certainly has a place, even amongst high level athletes, this doesn't mean it's optimal during all periods of the training (or competitive) cycle.

Growth hormone levels rise, this helps preserve muscle mass and shifts fuel metabolism to Intermittent burning. Furthermore, insulin sensitivity in the muscles increases, this sets the perfect storm for lean muscle gains. By having improved insulin sensitivity, you can better direct carbs into your muscle stores and away from fat storage.

Testosterone is also boosted during fasting. Now if you were to eat first thing in the morning, you would miss out on these incredible benefits. As well, cortisol peaks in the morning. Eating with elevated levels of cortisol can trigger post meal hunger. This is why many people find it much easier to control their cravings when they utilize intermittent fasting. Now on the other hand, fasting for long periods of time is far from ideal. Fasting for 20+ hours will deplete liver glycogen shifting you into a catabolic state. This is when training performance may suffer and muscle building will be impaired.

We want to optimize catabolic and anabolic activity to support a lean and highly muscular physi□ue and get the best intermittent fasting results possible. This means that we want to withstand enough time in the fasted state to experience heightened growth hormone levels, improved insulin sensitivity and increased fat mobilization without becoming too catabolic. Therefore I recommend keeping the fasting length in the ball park of 16 hours. Some people will prefer longer fasts and other people will prefer shorter fasts.

Practical benefits of intermittent fasting include less time spent preparing, eating, and cleaning up after meals (versus a diet of six small meals a day, for example), and its flexibility. You may only need to plan for two meals and they can be larger portions. The major guidelines for the 16:8 fasting rely on the timing of meals and not exactly which foods you need to eat.

Intermittent fasting doesn't re□uire calorie or macro tracking, but can be used in conjunction with any healthy diet pattern you already follow. For those who struggle with mindless snacking throughout the day or boredom eating at night, having a strict eating schedule can prevent those unnecessary calories that can lead to weight gain.

With Intermittent fasting, eating becomes a reward. If you're running on an empty stomach throughout a chunk of your day, when you break the fast that turns into a psychological and, of course, physiological reward. Whatever you do before you break the fast gets reinforced by delicious food. No one ever talks about this, but for me, it's one of the most obvious reasons intermittent fasting is helpful. There may even be are some hormonal signaling benefits here, too, though they are, to my lay knowledge, unproven.

In addition, fasting helps you reprogram your brain. When you make a conscious effort to not eat at certain times of the day, particularly when others around you are tackling those donuts and bagels brought in by kind co-workers, you begin to decondition habits you've built up over a lifetime. You undo pavlovian responses. Over time, Intermittent fasting can mean you're able to walk by the free donuts and not think twice about it.

Since you're starting a new diet with 16:8 Intermittent fasting, fasting can give you some time to figure out how to make the fasting work - e.g. what to eat when you do get to eat. The conditioning and association aspect can also be helpful as you'll be breaking your fast with high-protein meals, making those meals more satisfying and satiable. In other words, you might find it easier to comply with the high-protein requirements because you're fasting.

16:8 intermittent fasting reduces your cognitive load for making decisions. When you're cutting calories, not eating is easier than eating a little less at every meal. Decisions are hard. Willpower is fleeting. However, if you've made the decision in advance not to eat during certain times of the day, well, you don't have to think about whether or not to eat those donuts. The decision has already been made, which is to say there's no decision to make. It's like chunking for your "to eat or not" decision. You'll be less distracted. You won't have to use your willpower. Your brain will thank you. And no, fasting or lifting heavy weights for a few sets is not going to waste your muscle. But the key is to keep your fasts a reasonable length (16 is totally reasonable).

Does Fasting Agree With Your Natural Instincts?

We've all been told that breakfast is the most important meal of the day and that we should eat light at night if we want to be lean and healthy. It still pains me to see how widespread this mythical nonsense is.

The truth of the matter is that humans have evolved to eat sparingly during the day and feast at night. In fact, breakfast is a relatively recent phenomenon. The idea that breakfast is the most important meal of the day has largely been pushed by cereal companies to increase the sales of their food products.

If you look at the ancient Greeks, arguably the finest people to ever live, physically and mentally, they ate but two meals per day (lunch and dinner). They were obsessed with digestion and to eat more often was considered a form of gluttony.

By skipping breakfast and eating big and satisfying meals, fastinging becomes far more enjoyable than ever before. This is because you are eating in accordance with your genetic code, not against it.

Most people tend to function best fasting during the day and eating more food later in the day. This is because fasting triggers the sympathetic nervous system, this keeps you alert, focused and energetic. When you eat big meals, especially ones with carbs, you shift your body into the parasympathetic mode.

This makes you feel relaxed and sleepy. By utilizing Intermittent fasting your work productivity during the day goes through the roof and you have deep, restful sleeps at night.

But won't eating big at night cause me to store fat? You're kidding right? The only way to experience true net fat gain is to be in a calorie surplus. This is when you take in more calories than your body re□uires. As a result, your body stores the excess calories in your fat and muscle stores.

So as long as you're eating less calories than your body re□uires then you'll be experiencing net fat loss each day, even if you eat a giant meal before going to bed.

Best Foods to Eat While Intermittent Fasting

Okay, so you have the time windows for when you can chow down, but you're probably wondering what to eat during your journey. I've rounded up 20 of the best foods to create the ultimate Intermittent fasting food guide that will help prevent nutrient shortfalls.

Water. One of the most important aspects of maintaining a healthy eating pattern while intermittent fasting is to promote hydration. As we go without fuel for 12-16 hours, our body's preferred energy source is the sugar stored in the liver, also known as glycogen. As this energy is burned, so disappears a large volume of fluid and electrolytes. Drinking 8+ cups of water per day will prevent dehydration and also promote better blood flow, cognition, and muscle and joint support during your Intermittent fasting regimen.

Coffee. What about a warm cup of Joe? Will a daily Starbucks run break the fast? It's a common question among newbie Intermittent fasters, but worry not: coffee is allowed. Because in its natural state coffee is a calorie-free beverage, it can even technically be consumed outside a designated feeding window, but the minute syrups, creamers, or candied flavorings are added, it can no longer be consumed during the time of the fast, so that's something to keep in mind if you usually doctor up your drink.

Minimally-Processed Grains. Carbohydrates are an essential part of life and are most definitely not the enemy when it comes to weight loss. Because a large chunk of your day will be spent fasting during this fasting, it is important to think strategically about ways to get adequate calories while not feeling overly full. Though a healthy fasting minimizes processed foods, there can be a time and place for items like whole grain breads, bagels, and crackers, as these foods are more quickly digested for fast and easy fuel. If you intend to exercise or train regularly while Intermittent fasting, these will especially be a great source of energy on the go.

Raspberries. Fiber - the stuff that keeps you regular - was named a shortfall nutrient by the 2015-2020 Fastingary Guidelines, and a recent article in Nutrients stated that less than 10 percent of Western populations consume ade□uate levels of whole fruits. With 8 grams of fiber per cup, raspberries are a delicious high fiber fruit to keep you regular during your shortened feeding window.

Lentils. This nutritious superstar packs a high fiber punch with 32 percent of total daily fiber needs met in only half a cup. Additionally, lentils provide a good source of iron (about 15 percent of your daily needs), another nutrient of concern, especially for active females undergoing Intermittent fasting.

Potatoes. Similar to breads, white potatoes are digested with minimal effort from the body, and if paired with a protein source, they are a perfect post-workout snack to refuel hungry muscles. Another benefit making potatoes an important staple for the diet is that once cooled, potatoes form a resistant starch primed to fuel good bacteria in your gut.

Seitan. The EAT-Lancet Commission recently released a report calling for a dramatic reduction in animal-based proteins for optimal health and longevity. One large study directly linked consumption of red meat to increased mortality. Make the most of your anti-aging fast by incorporating life-extending plant-based protein substitutes like seitan. Also known as "wheat meat," this food can be battered, baked, and dipped in your favorite sauces.

Hummus. One of the creamiest and tastiest dips known to mankind, hummus is another excellent plant-based protein and is a great way to boost nutritional content of staples like sandwiches (just sub for mayonnaise!) If you're adventurous enough to make your own, don't forget the secret to the perfect recipe is ample garlic and tahini.

Wild-Caught Salmon. If your goal is to be a member of the centenarian club, you might want to read up on the Blue Zones. These five geographical regions in Europe, Latin America, Asia, and the U.S. are well known for dietary and lifestyle choices linked to extreme longevity. One commonly consumed food across these zones is salmon, which is high in brain-boosting omega-3 Intermittentty acids EPA and DHA.

Soybeans. As if we needed another excuse to splurge for an appetizer at the sushi bar, isoflavones, one of the active compounds in soybeans, have demonstrated to inhibit UVB induced cell damage and promote anti-aging. So, next time you host a dinner party in, impress your guests with a delicious recipe featuring soybeans!

Multivitamins. One of the proposed mechanisms behind why IF leads to weight loss is due to the fact that the individual simply has less time to eat and therefore eats less. While the principle of energy in versus energy out holds true, something that isn't often discussed is the risk of vitamin deficiencies while in a caloric deficit. Though a multivitamin is not necessary with a balanced fasting of plenty of fruits and vegetables, life can get hectic, and a supplement can help fill the gaps.

Smoothies. If a daily supplement doesn't sound appealing, try springing for a double dose of vitamins by creating homemade smoothies packed with fruits and vegetables. Smoothies are a great way to consume multiple different foods, each uniuely packed with different essential nutrients. Buying frozen can help save money and ensure ultimate freshness.

Vitamin D Fortified Milk. The recommended intake of calcium for an adult is 1,000 milligrams per day, or in plain speak, 3 cups of milk per day. With a reduced feeding window, opportunities to drink this much might be scarce, and so it is important to prioritize high calcium foods. Vitamin D fortified milk enhances the body's absorption of calcium and will help to keep bones strong. To boost daily calcium intake, you can add milk to smoothies or cereal, or even just drink it with meals. If you're not a fan of the beverage, non-dairy sources high in calcium include tofu and soy products, as well as leafy greens like kale.

Red Wine. A glass of wine and a night of beauty sleep may keep heads turning, as the polyphenol found in grapes has distinct anti-aging effects. Humans are known to have one of the enzyme classes SIRT-1, which is thought to act upon resveratrol in the presence of a caloric deficit to enhance both insulin sensitivity and longevity.

Blueberries. Don't let their miniature size fool you: Blueberries are proof that good things come in small packages! Studies have shown that longevity and youthfulness is a result of anti-oxidative processes. Blueberries are a great source of antioxidants and wild blueberries are even one of the highest sources of antioxidants. Antioxidants help rid the body of free radicals and prevent widespread cellular damage.

Papaya. During the final hours of your fast, you'll likely start to feel the effects of hunger, especially as you first start Intermittent fasting. This "hanger" may, in turn, cause you to overeat in large quantities, leaving you feeling bloated and lethargic minutes later. Papaya possesses a unique enzyme called papain that acts upon proteins to break them down. Including chunks of this tropical fruit in a protein-dense meal can help ease digestion, making any bloat more manageable.

Nuts. Make room on the cheese board for a mixed assortment, because nuts of all varieties are known to rid body fat and lengthen your life. A prospective trial published in the British Journal of Nutrition even associated nut consumption with a reduced risk of cardiovascular disease, type 2 diabetes, and overall mortality.

Ghee. Of course, you've heard a drizzle of olive oil has major health benefits, but there are plenty of other oil options out there you can use, too. You don't want to heat an oil you're cooking with beyond its smoke point, so next time you're in the kitchen whipping up a stir-fry, consider using ghee as your oil of choice. Basically just clarified butter, it has a much higher smoke point - making it a great choice for hot dishes.

Homemade Salad Dressing. Just like your grandmother kept her cooking wholesome and simple, so should you when it comes to salad dressings and sauces. When we opt to make our own simple dressings, unwanted additives and extra sugar are avoided. In fact, sugar might be accelerating the aging process more than any other ingredient by degrading cross-linkages of collagen fibers in our skin.

Branch Chain Amino Acid Supplement. A final approved supplement is the BCAA. While this muscle-building aid is most beneficial for the individual who enjoys fasted cardio or hard workouts at the crack of dawn, it can be consumed all throughout the day (fasting or not) to prevent the body from going into a catabolic state and preserve lean muscle mass. Note: If you choose to follow a vegan diet pattern, this supplement may be off limits, as most are sourced from duck feathers.

Foods To Avoid

Fats & Oils – Lard, coconut oil, butter or mayonnaise in excess.

Beverages – Alcohol, aerated and sweetened beverages, packaged fruit juices.

With so many veggies, fruits, spices, and herbs in hand, why not cook something delicious yet low in calories

Common Mistakes People Make While Intermittent Fasting

Before changing the way you eat and altering your fasting in any significant way, please speak with a health professional to make sure it's the best decision for you.

So your friend lost 15 pounds, and your dad can't stop raving about the blood sugar-regulating merits of intermittent fasting. You've reviewed the how-to manual and carved out a routine, but for some reason, you haven't seen any benefits. I've compiled some of the biggest mistakes you're likely making in your Intermittent fasting regimen.

1. You're jumping into intermittent fasting too fast.

The biggest reason most diets fail is because they're such an extreme departure from our normal, natural way of eating that they often feel impossible to maintain. Just a thought, but if you're new to it and are accustomed to eating every two hours on the hour, maybe don't throw yourself into a hard-core 24-hour-fast from hell. If you're adamant about the concept of fasting, start with a beginners 16/8 method where you're fasting for 16 hours per day and eating within the 8-hour window. That's probably pretty close to what you're used to doing, and who knows, it might be the only sustainable way to follow along.

2. You're choosing the wrong plan for your lifestyle.

Again, don't set yourself up for misery by signing up for something you know is going to cramp your style. If you're a night owl, don't plan to start your fast at 6 p.m. If you're a daily gym-goer who Instagrams their WOD every morning and aren't willing to sacrifice your daily spin, don't choose a plan that severely restricts calories a few days a week. You have to do you if you want any habit to stick.

3. You're eating too much during the eating window.

This one is the most common trap I would expect to see people fall into. If you've chosen a particularly restrictive regimen that's left you hungry for hours of the day, the moment the clock says "it's time to eat," you're likely to go a wee bit overboard. Research suggests restrictive fastings often don't work because we tend to become so emotionally (and physically) starved that when we do allow ourselves to eat, we go hog wild and overeat in a fit of deprivation. Any fasting that has you preoccupied with your next meal is a recipe for a binge so make sure you're not allowing yourself to feel unnecessarily hungry for long periods of time.

4. You're not eating enough during the eating window.

Yep, not eating enough is also legit cause of weight gain, and I'll tell you why. In addition to setting yourself up for a rebound similar to what we discussed with the last common IF mistake, not eating enough cannibalizes your muscle mass, causing your metabolism to slow. Without that metabolic muscle mass, you may be sabotaging your ability to maintain (never mind to lose) fat in the future. The challenge with IF is that because you're eating according to some arbitrary temporal rules, rather than listening to your body's innate cues, it's really difficult to know your true needs. If you're adamant about doing the fasting, be sure to speak to a registered dietitian to help you assess and meet your nutrient needs safely.

5. You're ignoring the 'what' in favor of the 'when'.

It is a time-centered diet, and most of the "plans" don't give any explicit rules about the types of food to eat during your "eating window." But that's not an excuse to subsist on a diet of French fries, milkshakes, and beer. Fasting isn't magic. In addition to some small metabolic advantages, its primary impact on weight loss (if it even has one) is largely based on the fact that you're limiting your number of eating hours and therefore reducing opportunities for calorie consumption.

Unfortunately, that effect can be quickly undone if you choose the wrong kinds of foods. Shift your perspective from the idea of treating yourself during your limiting "feasting" hours to getting in the most nutrient-dense, nourishing foods during those times. We recommend ensuring every meal or snack has a combination of satiating fiber, protein, and good fats to help carry you through your fasting phase.

6. You're not drinking enough.

Your Intermittent fasting regimen might have you refraining from food, but water should always be nearby, especially since you're missing out on the hydration you often get from foods like fruits and veggies. Dehydration can lead to muscle cramps, headaches, and exacerbate hunger pangs, so always make sure you're sipping H2O between (and during) feasts.

Followed all the rules and still struggling? It's not you; it's likely the fasting. Research suggests that Intermittent fasting has a 31 percent dropout rate, while research on fastings in general suggests that as much as 95 percent of diets fail. Try to focus more on what your body tells you, rather than what the clock says, and you're much more likely to get the nutrition your body needs.

Tea and Intermittent Fasting: The Perfect Match

If you're trying to stick to a new Intermittent fasting plan, you're going to want to see what we've learned about tea. Not only can tea make your fasting experience more enjoyable and manageable, but it will actually make your Intermittent fasting more effective.

Considered to be a health elixir in many ancient cultures, this simple drink is a powerhouse enhancer for your intermittent fasting lifestyle. You know all those incredible proven benefits you can get from intermittent fasting? Well, drinking the right kind of tea will actually increase the health benefits you experience.

Read on to discover the documented benefits that drinking tea can unlock for you, which teas you should be drinking, and also how much. Cheers!

How Tea Enhances the Benefits of Intermittent Fasting

1. Dramatically reduces hunger pangs

Especially in the first couple of weeks of Intermittent fasting, it can be very normal to experience hunger pangs. Please know, this is not because intermittent fasting causes any kind of starvation.

Those hunger pangs are simply a function of the fact that your system is spoiled and used to being fed every few hours. But remember, your body doesn't actually move from the "fed" state to the "fasted" state until approximately 4 hours after you've had your last meal. You don't want to give up on one of the most potentially beneficial eating plans around just because of a growling tummy, right?

Tea to the rescue! It's not just something to fill your belly. Green tea catechins have been proven to lower your ghrelin levels. What's ghrelin, you ask? Ghrelin is a hormone known as the "hunger hormone," and it is the primary culprit of those annoying hunger pangs. For many of us, lifestyle, environmental and biological stressors can lead to a hormone imbalance which will actually set off hunger pangs that have nothing to do with a true need to eat. Normalizing your ghrelin levels will alleviate this problem and help you adapt to intermittent fasting with minimal discomfort. Now that's a fast fix.

2. Aids in weight loss

Green tea in particular has been proven time and time again to be a successful aid in reducing body fat and LDL cholesterol. This goes above and beyond mere weight loss - these are true long-term health benefits.

The catechins in green tea seem to be particularly effective in burning visceral abdominal Intermittent, which is the most unhealthy (and potentially dangerous!) Intermittent that your body stores. In fact, studies have shown that green tea can aid in reducing waist size without changing body weight.

The other way tea can aid weight loss is because caffeine has actually been proven to increase your body's production of ketones. This means you'll slide into a Intermittent-burning mode even sooner.

3. Improves Autophagy (Promotes Anti-Aging)

Auto what? Your body relies on a process called "autophagy" to clear out old and damaged tissues and cells. You can think of it as housecleaning for your body on a cellular level. Autophagy is necessary to maintain muscle mass, reduce the progression of age-related diseases, and maintain mental health and function.

When you fast and give your body a break from the constant effort of digesting food, it is able to focus more energy on the repair functions of autophagy. Even better, drinking tea has been found to enhance the rate of autophagy in your body. This enhanced autophagy is the scientific reason behind why both tea and intermittent fasting have been linked to anti-aging.

4. Boosts detoxification

What makes tea such a unique substance is the polyphenols contained in tea leaves. Polyphenols are antioxidants that battle free radicals found in your body and have powerful detoxification properties. Ingesting polyphenols can help you experience improved gut health and digestion, healthier skin, sustained energy, improved mental clarity, a stronger immune system and reduced stress.

Tea is hands-down the richest source of polyphenols found in nature, but you do need to make sure you are getting them in sufficient quantity to experience these detoxification benefits.

Teas That Enhance Intermittent Fasting

The word "tea" often gets thrown around in a general sense when talking about healthy drinks. But have you ever found yourself staring down the tea selection at your local coffee shop or grocery store aisle and feeling overwhelmed? Us too! Especially if you're new to tea-drinking, it can be daunting to figure out which type of tea you should choose! We want to help you break it down by highlighting the four types of tea which can be most beneficial to use as Intermittent fasting tea.

Green Tea

Did you know that green tea is considered to be the healthiest drink in the world, right after water? It's true. As mentioned above, the catechins in green tea are proven to aid in reduction of body Intermittent and LDL cholesterol. And since green tea contains not only these amazing catechins, but also caffeine, these two elements work together to boost your metabolic rate and ability to burn Intermittent.

In fact, one study showed that your daily calorie expenditure could increase by up to 4% by drinking green tea. When that increase is happening on a daily basis, it makes more of a difference than you'd think.

The green tea catechins are also potent antioxidants, which are thought to protect the body from cellular damage and inflammation. And don't forget what we mentioned above about green tea affecting your ghrelin levels, so you'll definitely want to grab a cup anytime you're struggling with hunger pangs or cravings.

Black Tea

Fun fact: black tea and green tea are derived from the exact same plant! The only difference is in how the tea leaves are processed. Black tea leaves are fermented, while green tea leaves are not.

While green tea has continually claimed all the attention of the health world, black tea is finally starting to get the recognition it is due, particularly because of its fermented properties. Most people don't realize that black tea is a very potent prebiotic, excellent for promoting balanced gut health.

The fermentation process means that black tea provides slightly less antioxidants than green tea, but it also means that black tea provides more caffeine.

This might make black tea a great choice for you, because caffeine can not only help give you energy if fasting is causing you to lag, but it also has been shown to enhance your ability to switch to fat-burning and increase the rate of autophagy in your body.

The compounds found in black tea have been linked to increased heart health, plus improved digestion and detoxification, and even reduced stress levels. Black tea contains something called methyl xanthine, which boosts your serotonin levels. Increased serotonin leads to improved mood and relaxation.

So if you happen to find yourself stressed about your new intermittent fasting regimen, or maybe a bit grumpy during the hours you can't eat, black tea might be your new best friend.

Ginger Tea

A tea with added ginger is an excellent option while fasting. Ginger is well known for its ability to soothe an upset stomach, but drinking it can actually reduce hunger pangs and cravings. Ginger also has the added benefits of improving your digestion and boosting your immune system. So you can be less hungry and stay healthier too!

Rooibos Tea

Known to be a potent detoxification elixir, rooibos tea is an excellent herbal option, for when you don't want the caffeine boost that green and black teas will give you. Legend has it that Cleopatra drank rooibos tea regularly for clear and glowing skin. She was on to something, because rooibos does indeed help the body fight off toxins and improve circulation.

Even better, rooibos also supports your liver in processing Intermittents and clearing them from the body. One study showed that rooibos caused existing fat to be metabolized faster and prevented new fat cells from forming. No wonder rooibos tea is considered to be a powerful addition to an Intermittent fasting plan!

Intermittent Fasting Myths

There are many myths about fasting:

"Breakfast is the most important meal of the day!"

We have all been told to eat breakfast. Unfortunately this is terrible advice. When you first wake up in the morning, your insulin level is quite low and most people are just starting to enter the fasted state, 12 hours after eating the last meal of the previous day. The worst thing you could do is to eat food, spiking insulin and glucose and immediately shutting off Intermittent-burning. A much better choice would be to push the first meal of your day out at least a few hours, during which you can fully enter the fasted state and burn stored body Intermittent. The very worst would be to eat a high carbohydrate breakfast, spiking insulin and glucose as high as possible; in addition to shutting off fat-burning for likely 12 hours, this will drive as many calories as possible into fat stores as well as providing further reinforcement of the burning of glucose rather than Intermittent. Also, high spikes of insulin and glucose always lead to large drops in glucose a few hours later, which triggers hunger (if you want to have hypoglycemia or low blood sugar and ravenous hunger, just eat a breakfast of pure carbohydrates and then wait 2-3 hours to see how you feel). Interestingly, many properly fat-adapted people aren't very hungry in the morning and have no problem skipping breakfast. This is appropriate, as throughout our evolution humans have always been hunter-gatherers and rather than eating a large breakfast first thing in the morning we would hunt and gather throughout the day, having a larger meal later in the day. I highly recommend mimicking this pattern by skipping breakfast and eating most of your calories later in the day (referred to as a 'reverse taper' of calories, with none in the morning and most in the evening).

"Eat small frequent meals."

There has been plenty of worthless advice here. We have been told to eat frequently to "keep your metabolism going" and "don't let your body enter starvation mode". This is all the exact opposite of the truth: in order to burn fat, you want to spend as much time in the fasted state as possible and get very efficient at living on stored body fat rather than caloric intake from constantly eating. Similarly we have been told to eat protein fre☐uently throughout the day in order to build muscle, and this is also not evidence-based. Yes you do want to eat an adequate amount of protein to build muscle, but eating it once a day is plenty.

"Fasting leads to burning muscle instead of fat."

Many people are concerned that if they start fasting they will either stop making muscle or maybe even burn muscle. This is not true. If this were true, humans would not be here today. In fact, growth hormone is increased during fasted states (both during sleep and after a period of fasting). Growth hormone might as well be called "fasting hormone", as it rises by as much as 2,000% after 24 hours of fasting. Growth hormone is highly anabolic (builds muscle), and is used in combination with testosterone by bodybuilders who want to simultaneously build as much muscle and burn as much fat as possible. Growth hormone elevates in fasting to help preserve muscle in times of fasting, and this makes sense. In our hunter-gatherer ancestors, if fasting and going without food made you weaker and slower you would never catch or find any food and you would die and humans would become extinct. In fact the opposite is true; while fasting, muscle is preserved or can even grow if you are doing resistance training (highly recommended). Also, people experience an increased level of focus and alertness during fasting thanks to the release of epinephrine and norepinephrine (earlier in our evolution this increased energy and alertness helped us catch prey when necessary).

"Your metabolism slows down when you are fasting."

This is completely false. A number of studies have proven that in fasting up to 72 hours, metabolism does not slow down at all and in fact might speed up slightly thanks to the release of catecholamines (epinephrine or adrenaline, norepinephrine, and dopamine) and activation of the sympathetic nervous system (sympathetic nervous system is often considered the "fight or flight" system, while the opposite is the parasympathetic nervous system or the "rest and digest" system). It makes sense that this fight or flight sympathetic nervous system would be activated during the daytime, when hunter-gatherer humans are most active and in the fasted state (looking for food), followed by parasympathetic "rest and digest" mode in the evening after eating a large meal.

"If I don't eat I will get low blood sugar [hypoglycemia]."

Studies have shown that healthy persons who have no underlying medical conditions, who are not taking any diabetes medications, can fast for extremely long periods of time without suffering from any hypoglycemia. In fact, almost all sensations of hypoglycemia or low blood sugar (in non-diabetics) results from eating a very high glycemic index carbohydrate food a few hours prior (blood sugar spikes, then insulin spikes, then blood sugar drops rapidly). However if you are a diabetic, especially if you are on any diabetes medications, you definitely need to check with your doctor before starting a fasting protocol. Some diabetes medications can lead to severe hypoglycemia when fasting (mostly insulin and sulfonylurea drugs like glipizide, glimepiride, and glyburide). Be sure to check with your doctor prior to starting a fasting protocol if you have any medical problems, diabetes or otherwise.

"Fasting is purely a religious activity."

Not really. Yes many religions do have fasting periods but you find a lot of holistic health practitioners promoting or using fasting as part of an overall wellness regimen, whether it is for cleansing or for weight loss.

"We must eat often to fuel our brains."

When it comes to children eating breakfast, research seems to suggest that children do better in basic school tests after they have had breakfast as opposed to when they skip breakfast. The question remains, does this same rule apply to adults? The research suggests Intermittent fasting does not negatively affect adults. For example, in studies where healthy young adults ate as little as 300 calories over a 2-day period, participants experienced no decrease in tests of cognitive performance (including vigilance, reaction time, learning, memory, and reasoning), activity, sleep, and mood.

Not only has research shown that short-term fasting doesn't impair cognitive function, but it also improves brain health in many ways:

- Generates new brain cells - Intermittent fasting has been shown to increase rates of neurogenesis in the brain. Neurogenesis is the growth and development of new brain cells and nerve tissues. Believe it or not, you can create more brain cells and therefore improve your overall brain functioning with Intermittent fasting!
- Reduces inflammation – Intermittent fasting has been shown to significantly reduce inflammation. Excessive inflammation is the cause of many chronic diseases that we face today including Alzheimers, dementia, obesity diabetes, and more.
- BDNF production – Intermittent fasting also boosts production of an important protein called BDNF. BDNF has been shown to play a role in allowing the brain to continue to change and adapt. BDNF helps to produce new brain cells, protect your brain cells, stimulate new connections and synapses while also boosting memory, improving mood, and learning.
- Boosts Human Growth Hormone (HGH) Levels – Intermittent fasting has been shown to naturally boost HGH levels to provide healthy anti-aging, repair, neuroprotective, and longevity benefits.

"Juice fasting is OK to do."

Now some people would say this is a fad and not really fasting. Also the spikes of insulin brought about by natural sugars found in the fruit can cause unwanted side effects when there is no other food present. I believe that juice fasting is okay when done in moderation and can be used as a stepping-stone to start proper fasting which is far more effective.

"Fasting will make exercising more difficult."

Research has shown that any effect that brief periods of fasting has on exercise performance is minimal, if any. In one study, researchers found that a 3-day fast had no negative effects on how strongly your muscles can contract, your ability to do short-term high intensity exercises, or your ability to exercise at moderate intensity for a long duration.

In another 2007 study, researchers found that performing 90 minutes of aerobic activity after a 16-hour fast was not associated with any decrease in performance or metabolic activity. The exception to the above is long distance endurance athletes and elite athletes who train with multiple workouts each day might see a reduction in time before coming exhausted. And where performance is the number one priority over body composition. But for everyone else the combination of fasting and exercise may be a potent way to lose body Intermittent and maintain muscle mass.

However, there are situations where fasting can have a minimal negative effect on exercising. This comes from fasting during prolonged endurance sports, like marathons or Ironman, where you are exercising continuously for several hours at a time. The studies found that elite endurance athletes were negatively affected both in overall endurance and perceived exertion when fasting.

The bottom line is, fasting does not negatively affect anaerobic short-burst exercise such as lifting weights, nor does it have a negative effect on typical "cardio" training. You should be able to work out while fasted and not see any change in your performance. However, fasting is not advised preceding long endurance events. It is also not advised for elite athletes whose training involves multiple workouts each day.

"By fasting for long periods we can reduce toxins in the body."

This not correct as medical research will tell you long term fasting can strip the body of many vital nutrients creating an array of associated problems due to the body's powerlessness to deal with infections. To keep your body healthy I believe fasts are best done over short periods.

"Fasting is only really suitable for medical reasons."

This one again is not true. Yes we have all done fasts before having a blood test or operation but when done correctly fasting has many other benefits.

"Fasting is too hard."

This is probably the main reason people don't try fasting because they are just not sure they can handle being hungry. However this is not true because with a positive mindset a one-day fast twice a week can be accomplished by most people and does actually get easier the more you do it.

What Is The Importance of Calories & Macros?

It's important to note that this intermittent fasting guide emphasizes proper nutrition. If you're eating a poor fasting and not paying attention to what you eat then fasting will do very little for you. So it's important that you emphasize healthy meals while being accountable over your total calorie intake.

That said, I have found that Intermittent fasting makes eating healthy easier than ever before. This is because you start to crave natural wholesome foods like animal protein and veggies. On top of that, you're only eating 2-3 meals per day so fastinging is a breeze, you barely even have to think about it.

With each meal you will have plenty of calories to work with, this gives you a ton of options for incredible and downright satisfying meals. In addition, it affords you the luxury to be able to eat out at restaurants without blowing your fasting. What's more, fasting makes it damn easy to incorporate treats into your meal plan without going over your calorie numbers.

So understand that as far as fat loss and muscle mass is concerned, the calories and macros matter. I recommend thinking of fasting as a way to make everything more enjoyable while also realizing some of the incredible physiological benefits that fasting provides.

How To Determine Calories & Macros

The following is the complete guide on how to calculate your calories and macros.

Step 1: Calculate Your BMR

Whether losing weight or building muscle, knowing your basal metabolism rate (BMR) is very important. Your BMR is the calories your body requires to maintain functionality while at rest. In other words, if you were in a coma, this would be all the calories you would need to survive.

The Harris-benedict formula is commonly used to calculate BMR but isn't very effective because it doesn't take body fat percentage or muscle mass into account. Instead, use the Katch-Mcardle formula to calculate formula:

BMR = 370 + 21.6 * lean body mass

Note: lean body mass is in kg. To convert pounds to kg, just divide your weight by 2.2.

Here is how to find your lean body mass (LBM):

LBM = weight - (weight * (body fat percentage/100))

To get an accurate reading of your body fat percentage and LBM, I recommend getting a DEXA scan.

Step 2: Determine Your Physical Activity Level

Assuming you're not in a coma, you perform some sort of physical activity every day. The ☐uestion is what level you fall under. To determine this, you must add an 'activity multiplier' (x1.2 – x1.9) to your BMR:

- Sedentary (little or no exercise): BMR x 1.2
- Lightly active (training/sports 2-3 days/week): BMR x 1.375
- Moderately active (training/sports 4-5 days/week): BMR x 1.55
- Very active (training/sports 6-7 days a week): BMR x 1.725
- Extremely active (twice per day, extra heavy workouts): BMR x 1.9

Once you have this number, you now know your total daily energy expenditure (TDEE) number.

Step 3: Determine Caloric Intake Based On Your Fitness Goal

Now that you have your TDEE, it's time to determine what your fitness goal. For most people, they either want to burn Intermittent or build muscle. It is very important that you know which one you want to achieve so you can properly calculate your caloric intake.

To lose body Intermittent, the main focus should be to reduce caloric intake. The more body Intermittent you have, the more calories you need to shave off your TDEE. Again, I recommend getting a DEXA scan to determine your body fat percentage. To build muscle, simply increase TDEE by 20 percent.

Step 4: Calculate Caloric Intake For Training & Non-Training Day

The last step for calculating calories is determining caloric intake for training and non-training days. When following 16:8 intermittent fasting diet, you will eat more calories on workout days vs. Rest days. This was purposely designed to optimize recovery.

Here are the e□uations for both days:

TDEE * 1.2 = training day caloric intake

TDEE * 0.8 = rest day caloric intake

Step 5: Determine Your Protein Intake

Now that you have a defined caloric intake, it is time to calculate your macros. Strategically consuming your macronutrients (protein, Intermittent, & carbs) is an integral part of the 16:8 Intermittent fasting fasting.

Of the three macronutrients, protein will usually be the highest ratio. Protein is the building blocks of muscles, so its importance is without question, especially after a strenuous workout. In addition, it helps protect muscle mass while dieting down and losing weight. Your fitness goal will determine how much protein you should intake on a daily basis.

When trying to shed body fat, research suggests that your protein intake should be about 2.3-3.1 g/kg (~1.1-1.4 g/lb.) per lean body mass. For example, if your LBM is 140lb (63.5 kg), then you should aim for 154-196 grams of protein per day. Any lower than that number and you risk losing muscle mass.

When trying to bulk up and build muscle, you should aim to get slightly less protein per LBM than Intermittent loss: 1.6-2.2 g/kg (~0.8-1.0 g/lb). So the same guy who has 140lb of LBM would be consuming 112-140 grams of protein per day.

While some think you need to actually consume more protein than this, that's really not going to help you unless you're on steroids or other muscle-building drugs. However, to maximize your bulking efforts, I suggest consuming as much protein as you weigh in LBM every day.

Step 6: Determine Your Intermittent Intake

Don't let these fad diets fool you. Fat intake helps regulate your hormones, so it essential that you get enough per day. For daily fat intake, aim to get 0.9 g/kg (~0.4 g/lb.) of LBM regardless of your fitness goal.

For 16:8 Intermittent fasting, remember that fat intake will be higher on rest days than training days. The reason for this is to maximize calorie partition. e.g., improved workout recovery, better Intermittent loss. To burn body fat, aim for the following fat intake per day: 0.9-1.3 g/kg (~0.4-0.6 g/lb.) of LBM. On rest days, increase that number by 30 percent. On training days, decrease that number by 30 percent.

To build muscle, your daily Intermittent intake should be around 20-30 percent of total calorie intake. Keep in mind that there are 9 calories for each gram of fat on rest days, multiply that number by 1.3 to get fat intake. On training days, multiply that number by 0.7 to get Intermittent intake.

Step 7: Determine Your Carb Intake

Carbs finish the macro equation. Carbs are essential because it provides energy and helps with muscle building, restoration, and recovery.

Regardless of your fitness goal, here is how to calculate carbs for your rest and training days.

Rest day carb intake = rest day calorie intake – rest day fat intake – rest day protein intake

Training day carb intake = training day calorie intake – training day fat intake – training day protein intake.

Intermittent Fasting FAQ

Who should not fast?

You should not do Intermittent fasting if you are:

- Underweight (BMI < 18.5) or have an eating disorder like anorexia.
- Pregnant - you need extra nutrients for your child.
- Breastfeeding - you need extra nutrients for your child.
- A child under 18 - you need extra nutrients to grow.

You can probably fast, but may need medical supervision, under these conditions:

- If you have diabetes mellitus - type 1 or type 2.
- If you take prescription medication.
- If you have gout or high uric acid.
- If you have any serious medical conditions, such as liver disease, kidney disease, or heart disease.

Won't intermittent fasting put me into starvation mode?

No. This is the most common myth about Intermittent fasting, and generally it's not true. In fact, some studies indicate that Intermittent fasting may even increase the basal metabolic rate (at least initially) and might potentially improve overall body composition.

Can I exercise during fasting?

Yes. You can continue all your usual activities, including exercise, while fasting. You do not need to eat before exercising to provide energy. Instead, your body can burn stored energy (like body Intermittent) for energy.

However, for long duration aerobic exercise, eating before exercise may increase performance. This is good to know if you're competing. Keep in mind that it may be important to drink fluids and replenish sodium (salt) around exercise when fasting.

What are the possible side effects?

There can be a number of possible nuisance side effects of Intermittent fasting. Here's what to do if you encounter them:

- Hunger is the most common side effect of Intermittent fasting. This may be less of an issue if you're already on a keto or low-carb, higher-fat fasting.
- Constipation is common. Less going in means less going out. You don't need medications unless you experience discomfort. Standard laxatives can be used to help.
- Headaches are common and tend to disappear after the first few times on fasts. Taking some extra salt often helps mitigate such headaches.
- Mineral water may help if your stomach tends to gurgle.

Other possible side effects include dizziness, heartburn and muscle cramps. Learn more A more serious side effect is the refeeding syndrome. Fortunately, this is rare and generally only happens with extended fasts (5-10 days or more) when one is undernourished.

Why does my blood sugar go up during fasting?

This is due to hormonal changes that occur during Intermittent fasting. Your body is producing sugar in order to provide energy for your system. This is a variation of the Dawn Phenomenon.

How do I manage hunger?

The most important thing to realize is that hunger usually passes like a wave. Many people worry that hunger during intermittent fasting will continue to build until it is intolerable, but this does not normally happen. Instead, hunger comes in a wave. If you simply ignore it and drink a cup of tea or coffee, it will often pass.

During extended fasts, hunger will often increase into the second day. After that, it gradually recedes; and many people report a complete loss of hunger sensation by day 3-4. Your body is now being powered by fat. In essence, your body is 'eating' its own fat for breakfast, lunch and dinner and therefore is no longer hungry.

Won't Intermittent fasting burn muscle?

Not really. During fasting, the body first breaks down glycogen into glucose for energy. After that, the body increases fat breakdown to provide energy. Excess amino acids (the building blocks of proteins) are also used for energy, but the body does not burn its own muscle for fuel unless it has to.

It would be a long stretch of the imagination to think that our bodies store energy so carefully in the form of glycogen and fat only to burn muscle when it is needed. In my experience with over 1,000 patients on various intermittent fasting regimens, exactly zero have complained that they have noticed significant muscle loss.

What are your top tips for intermittent fasting?

Here are the nine top tips, briefly:

- Drink water
- Stay busy
- Drink coffee or tea
- Ride out the hunger waves
- If people are not supportive of you intermittently fasting for health reasons, you don't have to tell them.
- Give yourself one month to see if Intermittent fasting (such as 16:8) is a good fit for you
- Follow a low-carb diet between fasting periods. This reduces hunger and makes Intermittent fasting easier.
- It may also increase the effect on weight loss and type 2 diabetes reversal, etc.
- Don't binge after fasting

How do I break a fast?

Gently. The longer the fast, the more gentle you might have to be. Eating too large a meal after fasting can give you a stomach ache. While this is hardly serious, people usually learn quickly to eat as normally as possible after a fast.

Isn't it important to have breakfast every morning?

Not necessarily. This appears to be an old misconception, based on speculation and statistics, and it does not hold up when it's tested. Skipping your morning meal gives your body more time to burn fat for energy. Since hunger is lowest in the morning, it may be easiest to skip it and break your fast later in the day.53

Can women fast?

Yes, but there are exceptions. Women who are underweight, pregnant or breastfeeding should not fast. Furthermore, for women trying to conceive, be aware that – perhaps especially for athletic women with low body fat percentage – intermittent fasting might increase the risk of irregular menses, and lower the chance of conception. Other than that, there is no special reason why women should not fast.

Women can have problems during Intermittent fasting, but so can men. Sometimes women do not get the results they want, but that happens to men, too. Studies show that the average weight loss for women and men who fast is similar.

Isn't fasting the same as reducing calories?

No, not necessarily. Fasting can reduce the time you spend eating and primarily addresses the question of "when to eat". Calorie reduction addresses the question of "what and how much to eat". They are separate issues and should not be confused with each other. Fasting may reduce calories but its benefits extend far beyond that.

Will I lose weight?

Most likely. It is almost inconceivable that you will not lose weight if you do not eat. In theory it's of course possible to eat more after fasting, cancelling out the weight lost. But studies generally show that people tend to end up eating significantly less overall. I call Intermittent fasting "the ancient secret of weight loss" because it might be one of the most powerful dietary interventions for weight loss, yet it has been mostly ignored by doctors and dieticians for a long time.

How much weight will i lose?

The amount of weight you lose with fasting is determined by how often and long your fasts are, what you eat afterward, and other factors. Fasting for 16-20 hours a day can help you safely lose 2-3 pounds of Intermittent every week.

While losing this much weight every week is great, it's how it makes it happen that's really cool. Losing weight with Intermittent fasting means that you will never have to count calories or plan and prepare several meals a day.

Conclusion

Intermittent fasting like the 16:8 diet can be an effective strategy for weight loss and exercise performance without re□uiring counting calories or tracking macros. The 16:8 diet can also decrease fat mass while preserving muscle, leading to lean gains. While more research is needed, it shows promising results for body composition, performance, and health related outcomes.

Once you are properly Intermittent adapted, intermittent fasting is actually easy, fun, enjoyable, and liberating - while making you leaner and healthier in the process! Let's say you are following the Leangains protocol. Breakfast every day during the work week is now just black coffee, how easy is that? No more worrying about what you are going to grab for breakfast as you rush around in the morning and struggle to get to work on time. This saves you a ton of time and work and effort and is literally a form of metabolic exercise in the meantime, improving your insulin sensitivity and strengthening your fat adaptation. This is a win in many ways. It also frees you to eat very large and satisfying meals in the evening, without feeling the deprivation of watching calories or restricting yourself. And on days where you skip breakfast and lunch, you will be amazed at how much extra time you will have when you don't have to worry about what to eat, where to get it, and when to find time to eat it. Your productivity will be higher as concentration and focus is higher in the fasted state, and you will have more free time.

Some Pointers

- Check with your doctor before initiating Intermittent fasting, especially if you are diabetic and on diabetes medications.
- You can generally take any vitamins or supplements you want while fasting as long as they don't have calories, but you don't need any supplements as you will be eating plenty of nutrient-dense foods every day.

- You don't have to worry about losing muscle from lack of protein during your fast, as long as you eat adequate protein at the meals before and after fasting.
- You will not lose muscle while fasting as long as you are exercising regularly, and I specifically recommend resistance training such as lifting weights.
- Following a LCHF (low carb high Intermittent) diet pairs nicely with Intermittent fasting, as both improve Intermittent adaptation a great deal.
- It is perfectly fine to exercise while fasting, either cardio or lifting weights (lifting weights is better for body composition and I highly recommend it for everyone, as this will further your goals considerably).
- Drink plenty of water and non-caloric beverages while fasting; coffee and tea in the morning make fasting considerably more enjoyable in addition to health and fat-burning benefits and are therefore highly recommended.
- Don't use intermittent fasting as an excuse to eat tons of junk food when you are eating - continue to eat responsibly, sticking with whole natural foods with high nutrient density and avoiding processed foods.

www.ingramcontent.com/pod-product-compliance
Lightning Source LLC
Chambersburg PA
CBHW070440290526
45791CB00005B/2053